Yoga for Men

A Beginners Guide To Core Strength, Flexibility and Better Health

Ryan Briggs

Introduction

I want to thank you and congratulate you for purchasing this book, "Yoga for Men: A Beginners Guide to Core Strength, Flexibility and Better Health".

This book contains proven steps and strategies on how men can do yoga.

Many people think that yoga is just for the ladies, but this book will show you just how beneficial—and manly—yoga truly is. You will find steps on how to perform basic poses and power moves that will not only get you started on doing yoga, but also even help you improve your performance in other sports and physical activities.

Contents

What's in this book?

Yoga for Men - A Beginners Guide To Core Strength, Flexibility and Better Health is written specifically for men who have never tried yoga before and are a bit unsure about it.

Any doubts you may have will be blown away when you see all the benefits that it can give you and discover that it is something that "real men" can do with pride. You'll wonder why nobody told you about it earlier.

It doesn't matter whether you are an athlete looking for an alternative to your normal training routing, someone who has never really done much regular exercise or you are somewhere in between. Whatever your starting point, this definitely the right book for you.

The book not only shows you how to do each pose step-by-step but it also has tips and photos all the way through. In particular, it addresses issues that many men encounter when they first start practicing yoga, including stiff hips, tight hamstrings and poor balance. You will also learn ways to tighten your abs and lower your blood pressure. What's more, you can do all this from the comfort of your own home at any time of day.

One look at the chapter list and you will want to get started straight away. In just a few weeks of regular yoga practice you will be able to see improvements and in a few months you'll be a new man.

Enjoy!

Chapter 1

Yoga myths debunked

Yoga has become a very popular form of exercise. However, many people have a lot of misconceptions about what yoga really is. Men, especially, have qualms about taking up yoga because of these common myths.

First, the thought of yoga conjures up images of people in difficult contortions. There are definitely poses that look like human pretzels, but they are just a few of a many of poses you will encounter in yoga. Anybody can do yoga, even if they aren't very flexible. Most poses have variations that you can follow that allow you to do a sequence successfully. Even seasoned pros can still do variations that challenge their unique bodies further.

You might have an injury or a physical issue which prevents you from doing a full pose. That's ok. It's just like any other athletic activity. If you have runner's knee, then you lay off from doing full marathons until you recover. Likewise, if you are more comfortable and faster doing a breaststroke over a butterfly in the pool then you choose the option that's better for you.

Next, what makes yoga different from other forms of exercise is the spiritual aspect. Many people think of yoga as a cult or, more politely, a religion. You might not be very comfortable chanting ancient Sanskrit prayers and having your instructor preach to you about being one with the universe when you just want to get a good workout. Try thinking of these peculiar acts as serving practical purposes. The chanting helps to regulate your breathing and warm your body up before practice. And the preaching is really not any different from the motivational speeches you hear at seminars or from the pep talks your coach gives before a match.

However, if you want to follow a more spiritual approach to yoga then by all means go for it. Just be aware that you have lots of options in this regard and that you can "shop around" to find an approach that works for you.

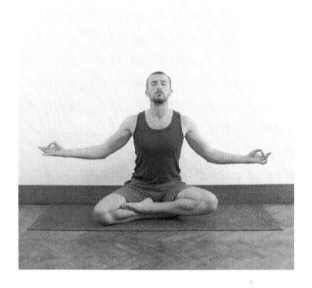

Lastly, it is definitely a myth that yoga is a girly activity that is not really very challenging to do. Historically, men have always practiced yoga. It's only in recent times that it has become mainly associated with Western women. The truth is yoga comes in different styles or traditions. There is yoga that is gentler. These are the yoga traditions that fall under the category of yin yoga. These involve less strenuous poses and you probably won't break a sweat from doing them. They are meant to revive and repair your body instead of putting stress on it. You will still get lots of benefits from doing such "easy" yoga.

The polar opposite, yang yoga, are styles that are more rigorous and will have you sweating buckets. You'll be moving faster and will be doing a lot of what you may recognize as body weight exercises. If you have ever seen a dedicated yoga guru in person, then you might have noticed his lean yet toned muscular physique. He definitely did not get his abs and biceps by simply sitting on a mat and chanting "Om" all day.

As with everything else, keep an open mind. Do not judge yoga simply by what the media or your friends tell you. Try it out for yourself and find out what bodybuilders, athletes, and trainers already know about it.

Chapter 2

Is yoga for me?

What are you looking for?

Men turn to yoga for a number of different reasons.
- Are you already an athlete looking for an alternative or supplement to your normal training routine?
- Do you look strong but lack core strength and flexibility?
- Are you overweight and not really into playing sport?
- Have you always wanted to have some muscle tone instead of being "that skinny guy"?
- Do you have an injury or disability that prevents you from doing many other forms of exercise?
- Do you just want something quick and easy that you can do in your lunch break and get away from the stress of the office?

Did you say yes to any of these questions? Whatever your reasons you'll find that there are many ways to "do" yoga and if you do your homework, you'll find one that suits your needs perfectly.

Different forms of yoga

The term "yoga" means "union" and refers to the union of the mind and body and also the union of the self with the universe / universal being. It originated in ancient India and is now practiced in all corners of the globe in many different forms. Traditional forms are still practiced in many countries and they often focus on elements such as devotion and connection with other through action.

The postures target different energy centers in the body called "chakras". Your instructor may refer to these at different times. There are 7 chakras and they are positioned in a vertical line from the base of the spine to the crown of the head. While this book does not go into a further discussion about chakras it is useful to know that each chakra is associated with different parts of the body. For example the first or base chakra is the energy center for the legs, hips, pelvis and lower spine. Postures that involve these areas stimulate the base chakra which then boosts energy and blood flow to them

Yoga practice increased in Western countries in the 1950's and 60's as people began to explore ways to connect with their inner souls. It was practiced by many "hippies" and became associated with them. In the following decades yoga became popular with middle class women as a form of exercise with the focus more on the physical benefits and less on the spiritual ones.

Since then yoga classes and schools have sprung up in many towns and cities around the world with countless forms and approaches. Some are centuries old while others have only started in the last few decades. The most common forms include:

- **Hatha yoga**

This form is popular as it uses slow-paced postures, gentle breathing exercises and relaxation to restore and strengthen the body, increase energy and calm the mind.

- **Iyengar yoga**

This form focuses on keeping the body in alignment. Postures are paused and held while in full stretch. It uses many props like yoga bricks and straps to help pull the body into alignment.

- **Bikram yoga**

This form uses many of the same postures as other types of yoga but it is performed in a room heated to around 100 degrees. The heat relaxes the muscles and the sweat releases toxins from the body.

- **Vinyassa yoga**

This is a more vigorous form that uses breath-synchronized postures.

- **Astingar yoga**

Here the focus is on constant, flowing movement through sequenced postures at a fast pace.

This book uses a mainly Hatha style approach.

If you are looking for a yoga instructor or class to join it is a good idea to ask how the instructor was trained and what form or style they teach before you sign up with them. You want to be sure that their approach will suit your nature and needs.

Why "do" yoga?

The simple answer is "Why not?" Once you get started you'll be wondering why no one told you about it earlier. Here are some of the many reasons to give yoga a go.

- It's cheap and portable

You can buy basic equipment or pay to attend a class if you want to and there is nothing wrong with that. However, you can also practice it anywhere you have the space at anytime you want. You don't have to buy specific clothes either.

- Yoga is not a competition sport

You simply focus on yourself. Don't compare how you are doing to the other people in your class. They have bodies and practices that are different from yours. Don't fret if the women in your class could gracefully float into a handstand while you are still struggling in downward facing dog. Naturally, women are more flexible, but flexibility can be developed over time. Likewise, don't scoff at the people who look like they are having a hard time. Leave out all judgment and negativity, and just focus on your own goals.

- It's ok to cheat a bit

If you need to put your hand against the wall for balance or sit on a chair to do a spine twist that's fine. You can even copy the person next to you which you were never allowed to do at school. (As long as they are doing it right of course.)

- Yoga can help reduce pain

If you suffer from acute or chronic pain you can ease it by reducing stiffness (especially in the back), strengthening the muscles that surround or support the painful area, or you can learn to relax enough to take your focus away from the pain and help you manage it better. Improving core strength and posture can also help alleviate some forms of pain as they reduce stress on the spine.

- You'll burn fat and gain muscle tone

A good yoga sequence will use nearly every muscle in your body. (See Chapter 5 for more about sequences.) A high powered yoga session is just as effective as a gym workout. Even the more gentle poses will burn some fat when you work just at the edge of your limits. As you get those muscles moving they will start to gain shape. When you twist your torso you massage your internal organs which helps them function better. Working on the pancreas, adrenal glands and thyroid will all help with weight loss. Muscles also burn more energy than fat so you'll start so see a difference on the scales too.

- It improves your breathing

You might feel that you can breathe quite well on your own and have been doing it all your life. But how would you like to run for the bus without getting puffed out? What about improving your lung capacity so you last longer in your next endurance race or breathing more clearly at night so you get better quality sleep? You can also use your breath to calm yourself down and gain more control over your body.

- Your doctor will love you

Have you been told you need to lower your cholesterol or blood pressure? How good would you feel seeing those numbers come down at your next appointment? Yoga improves your heart health and greatly reduces your risk of a stroke or heart attack plus it gives you extra stamina.

- Your partner will love you (more)

By improving your endurance, strength and breathing you'll also improve your sex life. You'll have much more energy and control of your body so you can pace yourself and last much longer. Plus with your increased flexibility just think of all the new positions you'll be able to get into!

- It gives you better balance

Yoga works on your balance both physically and mentally. The poses work both sides of the body evenly and give you more stability. This tends to flow through to your everyday life and you'll soon find more balance and improved perspective there too.

- Yoga makes you smarter

Well not exactly smarter but you will find that you can think things through more effectively. You'll have improved concentration and mental clarity as a result of the focus you've developed while doing the poses regularly. As you get fitter, your circulation improves and carries more oxygen to the brain and all your other organs so they all function better. Better focus also helps you to stay calm so you can think more clearly in times of stress.

Ryan Briggs

Chapter 3

Before you begin

Things you will need

- Clothing

Anything that's soft and comfortable (and decent) is fine. Just avoid clothes that have buckles or zips down the front as they may be uncomfortable when you lie on your stomach. Also think about how your clothes will move when you are upside down. If they are too tight they may restrict your movement but if they are too loose you might give others a bit of an eyeful of bits of you that you would normally not expose.

Yoga is generally done barefoot. You can wear socks but be careful not to slip in some poses. If you are in a group be mindful of other people's noses and pay attention to your personal hygiene, especially if you are prone to smelly feet.

- Physical space

At the very least you will need enough floor space to be able to lie down with your arms and legs out in a star shape plus a bit extra. Also check your overhead space. You don't want to take out any hanging lights or bash your hands on an archway. In a class, have at least an arm's length between yourself and the people around you.

At home or work, try to give yourself as much privacy as possible. Deal with any potential distractions beforehand and try to shut out obtrusive noise. You can have music on if you want to but make it something that you find soothing rather than something that will get you up and dancing. You aren't doing a zumba class!

- Optional equipment

You could spend a small fortune on accessories for yoga if you wanted to, but that's up to you. Some classes may require you to purchase a few basic items such as your own mat and a blanket or towel to cover yourself with during warm down. At home you may need a mat if you have timber or tiled floors (or smelly carpet that you don't want to put your face against) and you can use any old blanket or towel for warm down.

If you want to practice a form of yoga called Iyengar, you may also need to buy your own yoga brick to use as a support or a strap to loop around your limbs and help them move into various positions.

At home you can place a pillow or rolled up towel under you for cushioning or support as needed. The Iyengar strap can be easily substituted with a belt or tie. For example, loop an old tie around both feet and pull on it to help draw your torso down when doing a forward bend.

A simple dining chair is a very useful companion for many yoga positions. Place your hand on one for balance when learning to do the Tree pose or sit on it to help make the Spine Twist a bit easier. You can also use it to rest your feet on in some of the inverted postures.

Beginner's tips

- Precautions

We all know that we should drink plenty of water. This is no less true when practicing yoga. It is not only important to prevent dehydration in general but if you are dehydrated, chances are your muscles and tendons will be quite tight too.

It's not a good idea to practice yoga after eating a big meal. You'll be more sluggish and may get indigestion from all that twisting, turning and lying on your stomach.

Most yoga poses leave you feeling quite invigorated so avoid doing them late at night. However there are some poses you can do that actually help you sleep. (See Chapter 13.)

- Adaptations for injuries or health conditions

It is important to speak to your doctor if you have any medical issues before starting a yoga regime. Although it is generally low-impact, you can still do yourself harm if you are not careful. Find out what your limitations are and stay within them. For example, if you have arthritis or an injury in your shoulder you may not be able to raise your arm above your head and avoid the inverted poses if you have serious eye issues such as glaucoma.

Many poses can be adapted to suit individual limitations. Our friend the dining chair has helped many people with arthritis still manage a yoga routine. In fact some yoga schools run chair-based classes for exactly that reason. If you are unable to get much movement in your legs, you can still move your arms or simply do some of the breathing exercises. Some poses can even be done when lying in bed. It's important to look for what you CAN do rather than what you can't do. You'll find that many poses ARE possible and you'll find your self-esteem will get a boost every time you complete them successfully.

- Warm ups and warm downs

As with any form of exercise, it is very important to remember to warm up beforehand and warm down afterwards. This helps to prevent injury and also loosens the body up so you'll perform better. If you have particularly stiff or painful areas be sure to give them some extra attention.

A good warm up to use is the "Salute to the Sun" sequence as it is quick and uses the whole body. (See Chapter 5). However you can devise your own warm up sequence to get the bones moving. Try sitting on the floor with the soles of your feet touching each other and your hands clasped over your feet to keep them still. Then feather your knees up and down like a butterfly, pushing them a little towards the floor. This will open up your hips and warm your lower body.

Another move to try is to stand with your hands in the air. Reach up with alternate hands as though you were trying to grab something off a top shelf. Or hold your arms out to the sides at shoulder height, then keeping your arms in a straight line, twist back to first one side and then the other as far backwards as you can without straining your lower back.

To get your breathing going and clear your sinuses place one hand on your nose and use your thumb and middle finger to gently close your nostrils. Open one nostril and breathe in slowly. Hold the breath for a few seconds with both nostrils closed and then open the opposite nostril and gently release the breath. Then inhale through the second nostril and reverse the process. Repeat a few times. This exercise is quite simply known as Alternate Nostril Breathing and the slower and more controlled you can do it the better.

It's a good idea to have a short rest between poses, especially strenuous ones as that gives you a chance to catch your breath and it also allows your body time to store the energy you have just generated so you can draw on it at other times. You can use the Child's pose (Chapter 13) or Corpse pose (Chapter 4) for these rests.

If your back is troubling you, lie on the floor on your back and curl your knees up above the chest. Use your hands to gently draw your knees down a bit further but don't force it. Roll around on your spine and press your back muscles down and massage them against the floor. This is a great way to relieve back pain and stiffness when there is no one around to give you a massage.

After your yoga session, give yourself at 5 - 10 minutes to warm down. Lie in Corpse pose until your breathing returns to normal. At this stage, some instructors may talk you though a mental relaxation exercise. They can certainly help to reduce stress and improve mental clarity. It's up to you if you want to try something like that at home.

Yoga Principles

When doing any of these yoga poses, keep in mind some of these basic principles.

• KISS – Keep It Simple Stupid

Don't push yourself too much. A lot of athletes are used to pushing their bodies to their limits. That is good, but don't rush into a full pose without doing the necessary groundwork first. As the saying goes, "Don't try and walk before you can crawl". Consider it like sports training; you need to learn and practice the basic skills first before you can win competitions.

If you are used to endurance or strength training you may be tempted to push hard and do lots of mechanical repetitions to quickly gain muscle mass. However, to achieve a supple and balanced body you may actually have to *decrease* the strength in some areas as they could be causing tension or weakness elsewhere. You could even be restricting your circulation and adding to your overall stress level.

Instead choose some simple postures and be fully aware of your movements as you do them. Aim to work the whole body smoothly and evenly. You'll soon find that this approach will help you achieve greater flexibility in all postures and restore balance and decrease tension both physically and emotionally.

- Don't force it

Listen to how your body is feeling at the moment and adjust your practice accordingly. It's normal to feel a bit uncomfortable as you stretch at your limits but if you feel intense pain or discomfort, stop. Forcing a stretch too hard could cause you a major injury such as a snapped tendon. If you are in a class that is too hard for you, speak to the instructor so they can suggest some modifications. You can try to do the more challenging poses as you get stronger.

- Stay focused

Exercising at the gym can sometimes turn into a mind-numbing routine of reps and circuits. Your thoughts stray and you zone out so you don't really pay attention to your movements.

In yoga you actively engage the mind. You focus on your various body parts as you move them and try and visualize how they function internally. In doing so, you can clear your mind of distracting thoughts and stay in the moment. This time-out is why a lot of people find that yoga is a great way to de-stress.

- Breathe

Breathing is also an important aspect of yoga. The general rule is to inhale going up or lengthening and exhale going down or stretching further often pausing for a moment in between. So, as you look up in the Cat/Cow pose (Chapter 8) you breathe in and pause; as you look down and arch the back you breathe out and pause again.

If you are holding a stretch for a length of time, remember to keep breathing and not tense up. Each time you breathe out you can stretch a little further.

Proper deep breathing is important most especially in the inversion poses so you keep oxygen circulating your body and prevent you from passing out.

Use your diaphragm to control your breathing. If you aren't sure how to do that, place your hands on your sides just below your rib cage (where the "spare tires" sit). As you take a slow breath you should be able to feel that area expand outwards like a balloon. Also, breathe in and out of your nose rather than your mouth.

- Line up

Keeping your spine in alignment especially during back bends will help you avoid injury. Check your posture by standing barefoot with your heels and shoulder blades against a wall. Your hips should be in line directly above your feet with as much as your spine as possible touching the wall. Pull your chin back and lift the base of the skull back above the shoulders. Avoid hunching the shoulders. Instead roll them back and down.

Straighten out the arch in your lower back by tightening your abdominal muscles and rotating your tail bone forward. Try and visualize a bit of space between each vertebra.

Poor posture is one of the major causes of back pain, neck pain and headaches as it puts pressure on the nerves and leads to tight, knotted muscles.

Good Posture

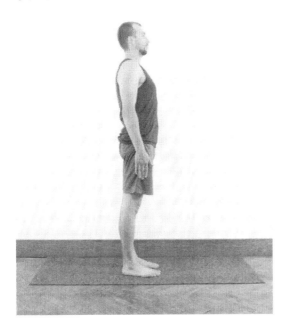

Bad Posture

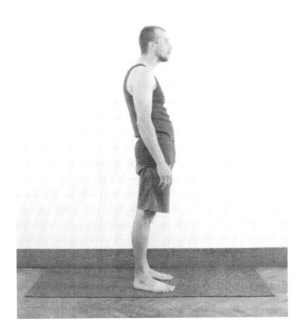

- Tips for forward bends

Forward bends do wonders for creating flexibility in the spine, hips and right down the legs; however they can cause discomfort in the hamstrings or lumbar spine or even cause a bit of damage if done incorrectly. Men in particular often have very stiff hips and tight hamstrings so they may find forward bends a bit challenging.

In a backbend, the vertebrae bunch closer together at the back of the spinal column and move apart in a small wedge at the front. This tends not to be a problem as there are fewer nerves and tendons on that side of the spine.

However, in a hunched forward bend the vertebrae bunch together at the front of the spinal column which can put pressure on or even pinch nerves or the spinal cord.

To avoid this, always start in an upright position and straighten the spine as described above. As you move forward, keep your tailbone tucked under and tighten your buttocks and abdominal muscles. Use your hips and pelvis to pivot forward and down instead of hunching your spine. Keeping your shoulder blades together will also help.

You may find that bending this way puts a strain on your hamstrings. If that is the case, then bend your knees to take the pressure off. When doing a seated forward bend you could even place a rolled up towel or pillow under your knees. As you become more flexible you can aim to straighten the legs.

Always remember to follow a forward bend with a gentle back bend and vice versa.

Chapter 4

The big 3

Foundation poses

In nearly every form of yoga you will come across these 3 basic yoga poses. They can be performed on their own or to aid transition between other poses. They may seem simple but they actually engage the mind and body completely so it's a good idea to get to know them straight away.

Mountain pose

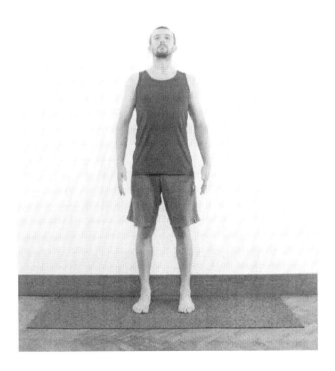

Benefits
- Works the whole body
- Promotes good posture and core strength
- Increases mental focus

The most basic yoga pose is the standing position. This is how most sequences begin. The pose does look like the practitioner is simply standing in place, but the mechanics are much more difficult. Many instructors call this the Mountain pose because you look like a tall mountain.

Step 1
Stand with your feet about hip width apart, your head facing forward and your arms loose at your sides.
Spread your toes out evenly on the mat so that you are strongly rooted on the ground. Your thighs and knees should be parallel to each other and facing forward. Bend your knees a little to reduce excess tension.

Step 2
Tighten the muscles in your thighs so that you are already working them just by standing. Tilt your pelvis forward, your tailbone down and engage your buttocks and abdominal muscles to hold the pelvis in this position. Aim to flatten the arch in your lower back. Check that your spine is straight and don't lean forwards or backwards.

Step 3
Roll your shoulders back and down and allow your arms to fall slightly away from your sides. Spread your fingers out with the palms facing forward. Check that your chin is parallel to the floor and lift your ribcage up.
Imagine that there is a string pulling you up from the crown of your head right through the spine as though you were a string puppet.
Hold this pose for a minute or so and feel the breath draw strength into your body.

Lotus

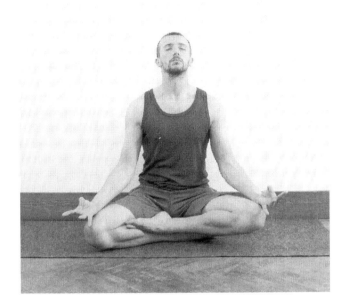

Benefits
- Improves hip and knee flexibility
- Tones leg muscles
- Improves posture
- Improves balance and focus
- Calms the mind

You will often encounter the lotus pose at the beginning of a sequence of sitting poses. Those who practice meditation find it a comfortable position to hold for long periods. You may like to sit on a cushion or folded blanket to manage this.

Step 1
Sit on the floor (or cushion) with your legs stretched out flat in front of you. Bend one knee and pull that foot toward your body.

Step 2
Gently lift and cradle that leg in your arms and push your knee

to the side. You can place your foot on top of or underneath the opposite thigh depending on your flexibility. Do the same to the other leg. The beginner's version is to have your feet underneath the thighs.

Keep your knees as low as you comfortably can. Having them too high may overstrain the flexors in your lower back, hips, pelvis and thighs. Instead, try sitting on a cushion and aim to drop your knees slightly below hip level if possible as this will allow your thighs to spread and relax.

Step 3
Place your hands in a prayer position with the palms pressed together in the middle of your chest. Alternatively, lay your hands on your knees with your palms up or down.

You can do the basic yoga mudra finger position with your thumb and forefinger touching and the rest of the fingers outstretched and the palms turned upwards. This finger position is also called the "Om" position and is believed to complete a circuit of energy flowing through the body.

Corpse pose

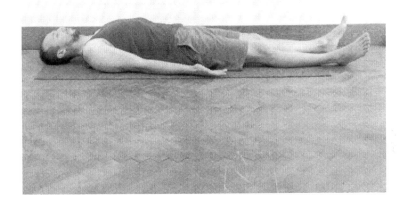

Benefits
- Improves posture
- Calms the mind and relaxes the body
- Reduces blood pressure
- Improves respiratory function
- Cools the body after a yoga session

The Corpse or Dead Man's pose is what you'd call "lying down on the floor". It is harder than it sounds, because you have to make sure that you are following the natural curve of your spine. So, there should be a bit of space between the floor and your lower back.

Step 1
Lay your hands by your side, away from your body with your palms towards the ceiling. Allow your fingers to curl naturally.

Step 2
Spread your legs just a bit beyond hip width and let your feet fall slightly to the sides. Close your eyes and focus on your breathing.

This can be used as a transition between poses and is also the last pose of a yoga session. It is essential for cooling the body down. Instructors who prefer to incorporate meditation would begin and end class this way.

Chapter 5

Putting it all together

Creating a sequence or routine

Doing yoga involves performing a series of poses (also called postures) in sequence. So, you will be transitioning smoothly from one pose to another in a somewhat choreographed dance. It might at first be daunting for you to have to memorize choreography, but you will easily get the hang of it. The sequences are logical and soon enough they will be instinctive to you. You might even be able to come up with your own sequences.

Many yoga routines incorporate a number of mini sequences and single poses. The routines usually follow a similar pattern. To begin, there are the warm up and breathing exercises. The 12-step sequence called "Salute to the Sun" is often used here as it works the entire body. Poses that work the legs, pelvis and lower back usually come first. Next are the sitting and twisting postures that work the back, abdomen and solar plexus area followed by the inverted poses that work the shoulders, neck and head. Finally, they conclude with some rest in Corpse pose.

Use the popular sequences below or create your own from the poses in the following chapters. Your personal routine will depend on the areas you want to address (hips, balance, tension release, etc) and also on the time you have available. Aim to go from gentle to more intense and then back to gentle again. If you don't have time to relax in Corpse pose, at least sit quietly for a few moments and allow your heart rate to return to normal.

Basic sequences

Salute to the sun
1.

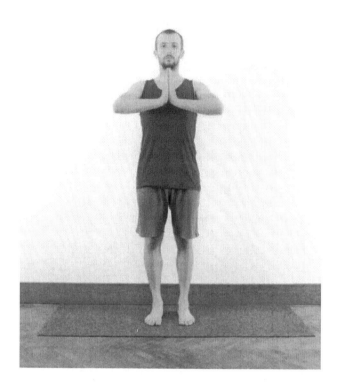

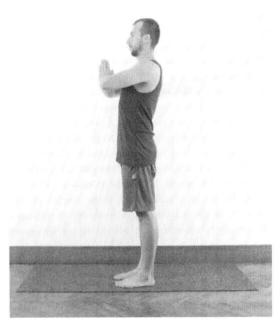

2.

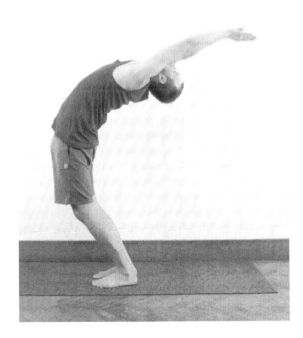

3.

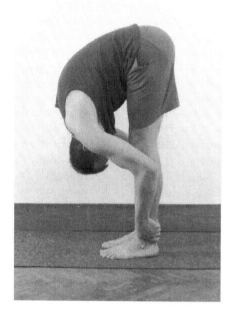

4.

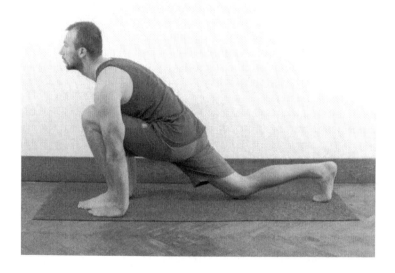

5.

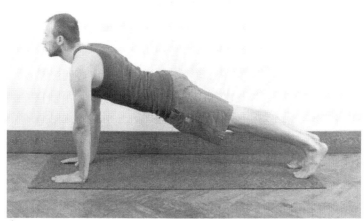

6.

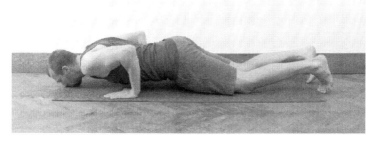

7.

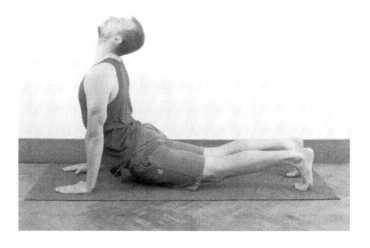

8.

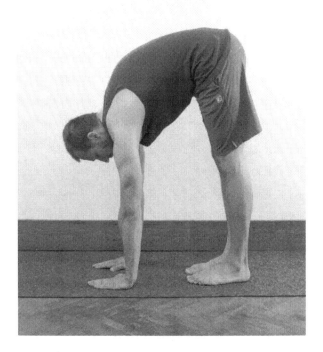

9.

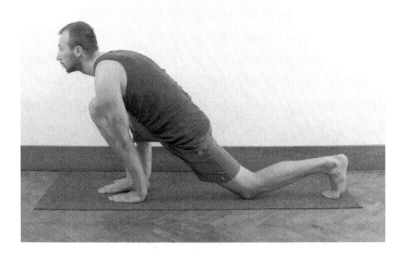

10.

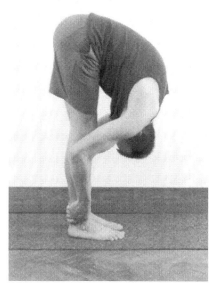

11.

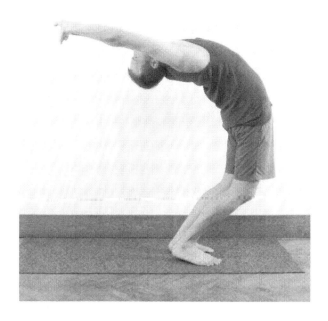

12.

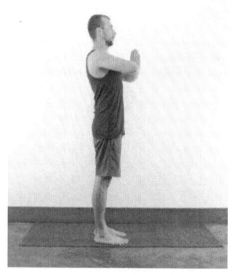

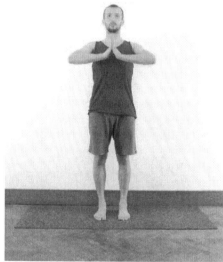

Benefits
In this sequence each step has different benefits and some steps are repeated.

- *Steps 1 and 12*
  - o Improve focus and awareness
- *Steps 2 and 11*

- o Open out the chest and fill the body with energy
- *Steps 3 and 10*
  - o Improve digestion by massaging the internal organs
- *Steps 4 and 9**
  - o Strengthen the ankles, knees and hips and increase their range of motion
- *Steps 5 and 8*
  - o Firm and strengthen the whole body
- *Steps 6 and 7*
  - o Expand the chest, tone the body, reduce fatigue and stimulate the nervous system, kidneys and adrenal glands.

The "Salute to the Sun" is a complete routine of physical fitness and relaxation in itself.

As the name suggests, this sequence is usually performed in the morning as it awakens the mind and body and gets you ready for the day ahead. It is sometimes called "Sun Salutation" or "Good Morning". It is ideal if you don't have much time as you can perform it 3 times in 5 – 10 minutes once you get used to it. This stimulates the breathing and circulation.

It helps to say the step numbers out loud and try and to match your breathing to the rhythm of the movements. At first you may find it awkward to move between the each pose. That's ok, don't worry about it. Just go at your own pace and work within your limits. Once your body loosens up you can aim for a smooth flow with no pauses between each step.

* "Low Lunge". In Step 4 you extend your right leg back and leave the left leg forward. However in Step 9 the left leg stays back and the right leg comes forward. This gives both legs an even stretch. An easy way to remember this is that you only ever move the right leg when going into this pose. The left leg stays where it is.

Step 1 – Mountain pose

See description in Chapter 4.

Step 2- Upward salute

Inhale and reach your arms up towards the ceiling then lean back as far as you can. Keep your arms beside your ears and reach out through the fingers to extend the stretch. Bend the upper back into a gentle arch and bring your shoulder blades together. Avoid bending the lower back. Breathe deeply and let your whole body enjoy the stretch.

Step 3 – Standing forward bend

Exhale and gently drop forward. Bend from the hips and keep your arms extended in line with your torso. Lead with your chest so you are not rounding your back. Keep bending forward until you can place your hands on the mat right beside your feet on either side.

If you can't reach the mat, then you can slightly bend your knees. Lift your chest and head up to look forward, then fold back to your legs again. Keep your hands on the floor in this position for the next few steps.

Step 4 – Low lunge

Inhale then, while supporting yourself on your hands, exhale and stretch your right leg out behind you with the top of the foot touching the floor. Lower the right knee to the floor then, leading with your chin, lift your head up. Bend the left knee and lower your chest to rest on the left thigh. Keep the left foot on the floor between your hands.

Step 5 – Plank pose

This pose is sometimes called the "Four-Limbed Staff". As you inhale, bring the left leg back parallel to the right. Drop your head a little so that your body is in a straight line or "plank". Avoid dipping or lifting your hips.

Check that your elbows are straight and your weight is balanced between your toes and your palms.

Step 6 – Salute with eight limbs pose

Other names for this pose are the "Caterpillar" or "Knees, Chest and Chin". The eight limbs are the chest, chin, two feet, two knees and two hands.

Exhale slowly and in one flowing movement drop your knees to the floor and sit back over your heels with your arms still stretched forward.

In the same movement and exhalation swing your chest forward and drop it to the floor between your hands. Then lift the tailbone up towards the ceiling and drop your chin to the floor. Hold without breath for a brief moment.

Step 7 – Cobra pose

As you inhale sweep your chest forward, up and back. Gently allow your head to drop back and look towards the ceiling. Lay your shins and the tops of your feet on the mat while keeping your thighs off the floor. Keep your shoulders relaxed and draw your shoulder blades together. Aim to keep your arms straight if you can.

Step 8 – Downward-facing dog pose

Next, tuck your toes under and plant your feet down on the mat. Exhale, raise your buttocks towards the ceiling and look back at your shins. You should be forming an upside-down V shape. Try to keep your heels down on the mat and your upper arms close to your ears.

Step 9 – Low lunge pose

This pose is a repeat of Step 4 but you are now stretching the opposite side. This time as you inhale move your right leg forward and place the foot down between your hands. Keep the right knee bent and close to your chest. Lower your left knee to the floor and also swing your chin up so your head drops back a little.

Step 10 – Standing forward bend pose

This pose is a repeat of Step 3. Exhale and bring your left foot forward so both feet are between your hands. Aim to keep both hands on the floor but bend your knees if needed. Look back between your legs and allow your torso to relax as gravity draws it down.

Step 11 – Upward salute pose

This pose is a repeat of Step 2. Inhale and look forward. Come up the reverse way you came down by lifting your chest and pivoting from the hips. As you come up, raise your arms above your head then back as far as you can while arching your upper back. Expand your chest out and enjoy the stretch through the whole body.

Step 12 – Mountain pose

This pose is a repeat of Step 1. To move back into it from the Upward Salute exhale and bring your torso upright while sweeping your arms out to the side and then down alongside your thighs.

Now inhale and bring your hands up in front of your chest in a prayer position while arching back slightly. Exhale and straighten up then briefly dip your chin to your chest and back up so you face forward. Drop your hands to your sides as you exhale and stand in Mountain pose. Stay there until your breathing returns to normal.

The "Warrior" poses

The concept of a warrior may sound out of place with yoga practice but the idea originated from the warrior gods Krishna and Arjuna. Now the name refers more to the idea of a spiritual warrior fighting against self-ignorance (a universal enemy). There are three warrior poses that you would often encounter when doing yoga. They are differentiated using numbers and can be performed separately or in sequence.

Warrior 1

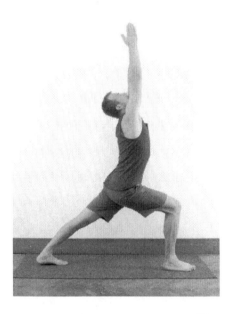

Benefits
- Helps to reduce pain from sciatica
- Strengthens and tones the muscles in the shoulders, arms, back and legs
- Improves flexibility in hips, knees and ankles
- Opens out the chest and improves lung function
- Improves stamina

Starting position
Stand in the Mountain pose and then lightly jump your feet apart about 3-4 feet.

Step 1
Reach towards to the ceiling and extend through your fingertips

Step 2
Swing the toes of your left foot towards the right about 45 degrees. Then swing the toes of the right foot to the right by 90 degrees.

Step 3
Keep your hands in the air then exhale and rotate your hips around so your head and torso face the right.

Step 4
Exhale and bend your right knee down over your right ankle. Aim to keep your thigh parallel to the floor.

Step 5
Slowly reach backwards and arch your spine gently as far as you can. Lift your chest up and look up at your fingertips while you hold the pose. Tighten your abdominal muscles to support the lower back. You should feel this stretch through your whole body.

Step 6
Keep your right knee bent and gently straighten your torso. Stretch your arms towards the ceiling and look out over your right knee. **Jump to Step 5 of Warrior 2 if performing the "Warrior" sequence.**

Step 7 (if performing this pose in isolation)
To come out of the pose straighten the right leg while keeping the hands in the air. Rotate the head and hips to the front followed by the toes. Stretch your arms out to the sides then slowly lower them to your body.

Repeat on your opposite side then return to Mountain pose.

Warrior 2

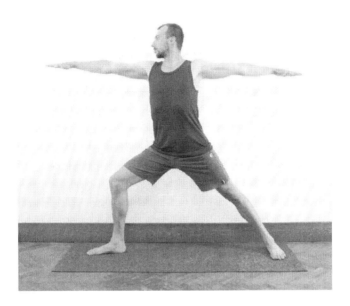

Benefits
- Strengthens and tones the muscles in the shoulders, arms, back and legs
- Reduces tight muscles in neck, upper arms and across chest
- Improves flexibility in hips, knees and ankles
- Stimulates abdominal muscles and improves digestion
- Opens out pelvic area and improves sexual function and overall energy

Starting position (if performing the pose in isolation)
Stand in the Mountain pose and then lightly jump your feet apart about 3-4 feet.

Step 1
Reach towards to the ceiling and extend through your fingertips

Step 2
Swing the toes of your left foot towards the right about 45 degrees. Then swing the toes of the right foot to the right by 90 degrees.

Step 3
Keep your hands in the air then exhale and rotate your hips around so your head and torso face the right.

Step 4
Exhale and bend your right knee down over your right ankle. Aim to keep your thigh parallel to the floor.

Step 5 (Sequence Step 7)
Swing your arms and torso around to the front keeping your right knee bent. Keep your head turned towards the right and avoid dropping the chin.

Step 6 (Sequence Step 8)
Lower your arms to shoulder height and stretch them out parallel to the floor. Extend the stretch by pushing your fingers outwards as far as you can. You might find that your right knee collapses inward as you do this. Keep your knee bent and above the ankle. **Jump to Transitional Step 1 (Sequence Step 9) if continuing the "Warrior" sequence**.

Step 7 (if ending the sequence here)
Straighten the legs, rotate the head and toes to the front then slowly lower your arms to your sides. Repeat on your opposite side then return to Mountain pose.

Transitional Step 1 (Sequence Step 9)
Keeping your arms extended, straighten the right knee then turn your head and toes to the front.

Transitional Step 2 (Sequence Step 10)
Raise your arms to the ceiling and step your feet together. **Jump to Step 2 of Warrior 3 if performing the "Warrior" sequence**.

Warrior 3

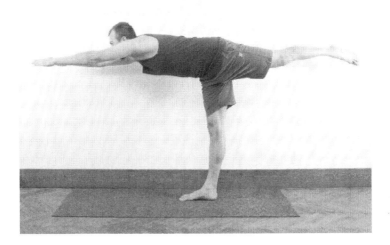

Benefits
- Improves flexibility in the hips, shoulders and ankles
- Strengthens and tones the muscles of the back, buttocks and legs
- Tightens the abdominal muscles
- Improves posture, balance and focus

Starting position (if performing the pose in isolation)
Start in Mountain pose.

Step 1
Raise your arms up and reach towards the ceiling.

Step 2 (Sequence Step 11)
Transfer your weight onto your right leg with your toes splayed out for balance.

Step 3 (Sequence Step 12)
Pivot from the hips and tilt your arms and torso forward and down. Raise your left leg backwards off the mat as a counterweight to your arms. Aim to stand on your right leg with the rest of your body parallel to the floor forming a T shape. Keep your chin up and look towards your fingers.
Keep your tailbone tucked under and use your abdominal

muscles, buttocks and hamstrings to hold the position. Extend out through your fingertips and heels. You can place your palms together so you look like an arrow shooting forward.

Don't worry if you can't get there at first. This is a very strong pose and it takes a while to build up the strength and flexibility to form it fully.

If you find yourself falling off your standing leg, try clawing your toes into the floor for extra grip. You may also bend the knee on your standing leg slightly until you can fully straighten it. Avoid overextending your knee to prevent injury.

Step 4 (Sequence Step 13)

To come out of the pose, pivot from the hips while you raise your hands to the ceiling and lower the left foot to the floor, keeping the elbows and knees straight.

Step 5 (Sequence Step 14)

Gently lower the arms to the sides, turn the whole body to the front and rest in Mountain pose. Repeat on your other side.

The "Triangle" poses

In either Triangle pose, aim to keep your chest parallel to the floor and your shoulders stacked on top of each other. Imagine that you are pressed between two sheets of glass, so your body looks like a flat triangle with one arm raised overhead.

The Extended Triangle is often taught early on as it is a basic pose with many benefits. However if performed regularly it should always be followed with the Revolved Triangle to strengthen the inner and outer thigh muscles evenly. This helps to give the knee greater strength and support.

Extended triangle

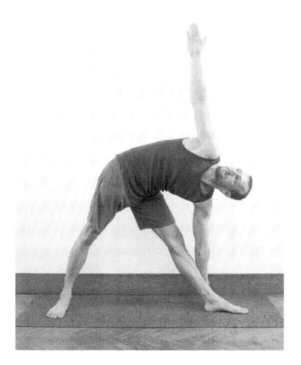

Benefits

- Improves flexibility in the hips, shoulders, knees and ankles
- Strengthens muscles in the lower back, groin, buttocks and outer thighs
- Expands the chest and improves lung capacity
- Stimulates the abdominal organs
- Improves balance
- Relieves tension in the body
- Reduces mild back pain and sciatic pain

Starting position
Stand in Mountain pose and then step your legs wide apart

Step 1
Stretch your arms out to the sides, parallel to the floor and extend out through your fingertips.

Step 2
Pivot your left foot about 45 degrees to the right. Then pivot your right foot about 90 degrees to the right. Turn your head to look out towards your right fingers.

Step 3
Slowly lower your right hand down and place it on the floor beside your right ankle or as far down on your right leg as you can reach. Use the muscles in your buttocks, pelvis and outer thighs to control the movement. Aim to keep the spine straight and the left arm pointed towards the ceiling.

Step 4
Keep your arms in line with each other and check that your left hip has not tilted forward. When you are steady, turn your head to look up towards your left fingers. Ideally your arms will be in line at a right angle to the floor.

Step 5
To come out of the position, carefully turn your head to look down at your right hand. With your arms still extended outwards, pivot your torso back into an upright position and continue to look out along your right arm. **Jump to Revolved Triangle Step 3 if continuing the "Triangle" sequence.**

Step 6 (if performing this pose in isolation)
Turn your head and swing your toes around to face the front. Inhale then exhale and slowly drop your hands to your sides and bring your feet together. Rest briefly in Mountain pose and repeat on the other side.

Revolved triangle

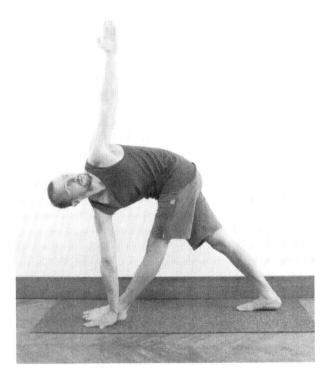

Benefits
- Improves flexibility in the hips, shoulders, knees and ankles
- Strengthens muscles in the lower back, groin, buttocks and inner thighs
- Expands the chest and improves lung capacity
- Improves digestion and relieves constipation
- Improves balance
- Relieves tension in the body
- Reduces mild back pain and sciatic pain

Starting position (if performing the pose in isolation)
The first 2 steps are identical to the Extended Triangle. Stand in Mountain pose and then step your legs wide apart.

Step 1
Stretch your arms out to the sides, parallel to the floor and extend out through your fingertips.

Step 2
Pivot your left foot about 45 degrees to the right. Then pivot your right foot about 90 degrees to the right. Turn your head to look out towards your right fingers.

Step 3 (Sequence Step 6)
Keeping your arms extended, swing your arms, head and torso around to the right so that your navel is now in line with your right knee.

Step 4 (Sequence Step 7)
Continue twisting your torso to the right while you reach down and place your left hand beside your right ankle or as far down on the right leg as you can.

Step 5 (Sequence Step 8)
Look up at your right hand and aim to keep your arms in line and at a right angle to the floor.

Step 6 (Sequence Step 9)
In one continuous movement, lower your right arm, swing your torso upright and turn it towards the front. Keep your arms extended at shoulder height and your head turned towards the right.

Step 7 (Sequence Step 10)
Turn your head and swing your toes around to face the front. Inhale then exhale, slowly drop your hands to your sides and bring your feet together. Rest briefly in Mountain pose and repeat on the other side.

.

Chapter 6

Keeping things in balance

Poses for stability, balance and focus

The concepts of focus balance and stability apply equally to our physical and emotional states. When our life seems out of balance we may feel as though we are being pulled in all directions and it can be hard to focus properly on everything.

By working to achieve good balance in the physical state we can also improve emotional stability and balance through a flow-on effect. Using a visual focal point in these poses helps us to develop our concentration skills and to block out unwanted distractions.

When you make these poses part of your regular routine you will soon find that you will have more control of your movements and also of your thoughts and actions.

Bird-dog pose

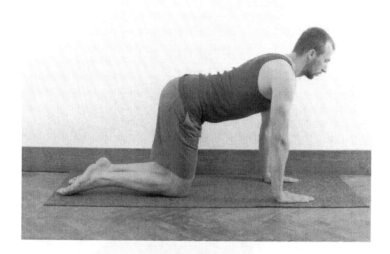

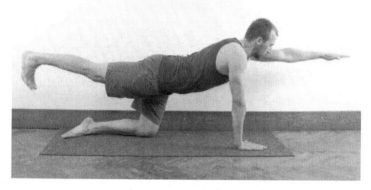

Benefits
- Improves core strength and tones abdominal muscles
- Builds upper body strength
- Helps to ease lower back pain and stiffness
- Improves left and right side coordination
- Increases hip and shoulder flexibility
- Builds up the strength and flexibility needed for the "Warrior" poses

Also known as "Hunting Dog", this pose is a great way to ease into the balance poses. It is also useful for those who find the standing poses too tiring

Starting position
Begin on your hands and knees with your weight distributed evenly. Check that your spine is straight, with your pelvis tipped slightly forward and a neutral curve in your lower back. Keep your head in line with your torso.

Step 1
Slowly extend your right leg back so that your knee is straight and the ball of your foot is on the floor.

Step 2
Shift your weight forward slightly and then raise your right leg. Aim to keep it parallel to the floor. Maintain your spinal alignment and breathe evenly.

Step 3
Once you have a steady balance, extend your left arm forward and bring the forearm alongside the ear.

Step 4
Point your left fingers and right toes to extend the stretch through your entire body. Hold the pose as long as you can.

Step 5
Lower your left hand and right knee back to the floor. If you experience discomfort in your lower back you may want to rest in the Child's pose. Repeat the pose using the opposite arm and leg.

Tree pose

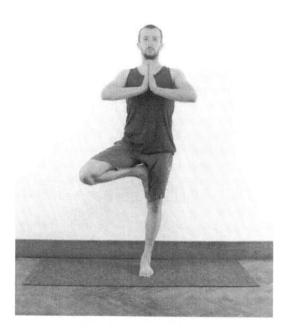

Benefits

- Improves physical and emotional balance and stability
- Tones muscles in the thighs, calves, abdomen and buttocks
- Relieves tension across the upper back and chest
- Improves concentration and focus
- Creates a sense of calmness and of being grounded

Starting Position
Begin in Mountain pose and transfer your weight over the left foot.

Step 1
Pick a stationery object to focus on in front of you around eye level. Keep your eyes fixed on that spot, raise your right leg and bend the knee. Grab your right foot with your right hand and extend your left arm out to the side as a counterbalance. Place the sole of the right foot against the inner left thigh. If you can't bring the right foot up that high, try placing it against the right calf instead.

Step 2
When you are steady press your palms together in front of your chest in a prayer position. Aim to keep your right leg out at a right angle to the body. Breathe evenly and hold the position.

Step 3
If you are comfortable and balanced you can try reaching your arms out the sides and then up towards the ceiling. Extend the stretch by reaching up through your fingertips and hold for as long as you can.

Step 4
To release the position, simply drop your right foot to the floor and bring your hands down into Mountain pose. Pause and repeat on your left side.

Eagle pose

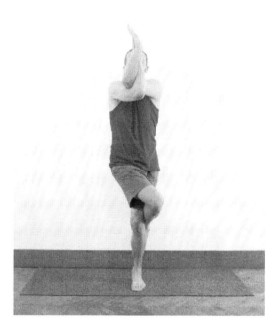

Benefits
- Improves flexibility in the ankles, knees, elbows and wrists
- Improves physical balance
- Increases ability to focus and concentrate
- Relieves tension

- Tones muscles throughout the body
- Relieves lower back pain and sciatica

Starting position
Stand in Mountain pose.

Step 1
Choose a stationary object in front of you to focus on. Squat slightly and take your weight onto your right foot.

Step 2
Keep your eyes focused ahead then raise your left leg and cross the left thigh on top of the right. Extend your arms out for balance if needed.

Step 3
Use your toes to hook your left foot behind the right knee. Splay the toes of your right foot out to help with stability.

Step 4
Raise your arms to shoulder height and point them straight in front of you parallel to each other and the floor.

Step 5
Place your right elbow into the crook of the left arm. Then point your fingers to the ceiling and raise both elbows so that your forearms are parallel to the floor. Your palms should be facing outwards.

Step 6
Rotate the wrists so that the palms now face each other. Push your palms towards each other as much as possible. Breathe evenly and hold the position as long as you can.

Step 7
Lower your left leg and drop your hands down into Mountain pose. Pause and repeat the pose on your opposite side.

Chapter 7

Love those legs

Poses for toning buttocks, thighs and calves

These days many of us have jobs that involve sitting or standing for long periods. Then we relax by sitting in front of the TV or around a table with friends.

Without regular exercise the muscles in our legs, buttocks and lower back become weak. This leads to poor posture and creates imbalances within the body.

The good news is that regularly practicing postures like these will strengthen your body and help to improve your overall health.

Chair pose

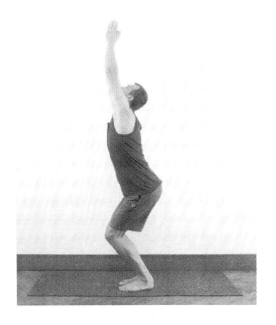

Benefits
- Improves strength in calves, thighs, ankles and feet
- Reduces tension held in shoulders, chest and thighs
- Expands the diaphragm and chest.
- Improves digestion
- Increases spinal flexibility and helps to reduce back pain

Starting position
Begin in Mountain pose.

Step 1
Inhale and raise your arms up either parallel to each other or with the palms together in a prayer position.

Step 2
Exhale and gently squat down keeping your thighs parallel to each other.

Step 3
Deepen the squat, lean your torso forward slightly and push your tailbone down towards your heels. Breathe into the position and try to lower the squat further on each exhalation.

Step 4
To come out of the pose gently straighten your legs, lower your arms to your sides and rest in Mountain pose.

High lunge

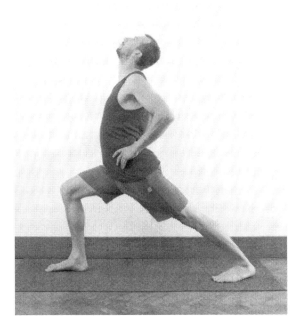

Benefits
- Tones muscles in the thighs, calves, groin and abdomen
- Increases flexibility in the hips, knees, feet, and shoulders
- Strengthens the lower back
- Boosts adrenalin and willpower
- Reduces tension in the shoulders, upper back, neck and chest

Starting position
Stand in Mountain pose.

Step 1
Place your hands on your hips and step your right leg back as far as you can with the toes tucked under.

Step 2
Bend your left knee and lower your pelvis towards the floor, pushing back through your right heel. Aim to keep your shin at a right angle to the floor.

Step 3
Tuck your thumbs firmly behind your hips for support then gently arch backwards lifting your chin and chest. Use your diaphragm muscles to breathe steadily.

Step 4
Slowly uncurl your neck and back while straightening your left knee.

Step 5
Bring your right leg forward and rest in Mountain pose. Repeat the pose on your opposite side.

Three-legged dog

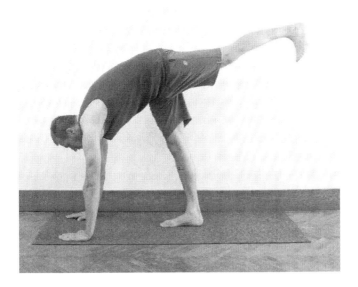

Benefits
- Tones the muscles in the buttocks, thighs and upper arms
- Increases flexibility in the hips, shoulders, wrists and ankles
- Reduces blood pressure
- Reduces fatigue and excess fluid in the lower legs
- Improves balance

Starting position
Begin on your hands and knees.

Step 1
Push your buttocks towards the ceiling then straighten your arms and legs. Keep your palms and heels flat on the floor and your head, tailbone and spine in alignment. This is the Downward-Facing Dog pose. (See Chapter 11.)

Step 2
Spread your weight between your left foot and both hands. Keep your knees straight then slowly raise your right leg as far as you can. Aim to keep this leg in line with your spine. Push

outwards with your heels.

Step 3
Slowly lower your right foot to the floor then drop back onto your hands and knees. If want to you can rest in Child's pose. Repeat the pose on your other side.

Chapter 8

Move your pelvis like Elvis

Poses to improve hip flexibility, sexual function and energy

Many of our vital organs and glands are contained within the abdominal and pelvic regions. When these areas become stiff or weak, the organs inside don't get the stimulation they need to function normally.

By regularly moving these areas in a targeted manner we can boost their performance significantly.

Cat / Cow pose

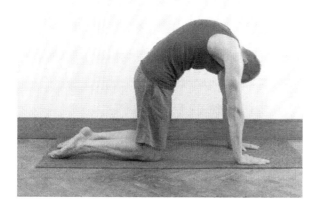

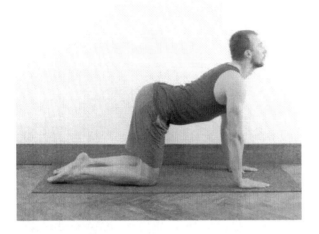

Benefits
- Improves flexibility in spine, hips and pelvis
- Strengthens and tones abdominal, neck and chest muscles
- Strengthens wrists, arms and thighs
- Improves digestion
- Stimulates adrenalin and sexual drive
- Improves sense of sexuality / libido

This sequence will prepare you for all the forward and backward bends you may do later on.

Starting position
Kneel on the floor then drop forward onto your hands and knees. Place your hands directly under your shoulders and your knees directly under your hips. Lift your chin and look forward.

Step 1
Take a deep breath and tighten the muscles in your abdomen and buttocks.

Step 2
Inhale and push your tailbone towards the ceiling without moving your arms or legs. At the same time lift your sternum and raise your chin up so that your head is resting on the back of your shoulders. Use your diaphragm to expand your chest and draw air deep into your lungs. Aim to create a strong arch along your spine and visualize a cat doing this stretch as it wakes up. Pause for a moment.

Step 3
Exhale and tighten your abdominal muscles while you push all
the air from your lungs. Use the muscles in your buttocks and
thighs to draw your tailbone back down and to tuck it under the
pelvis. Also push lower your chin so that it rests against your
chest and lengthens the back of your neck.
This the "cow" part of the mini-sequence. Hold for a moment
without breath.

Step 4
Repeat the sequence several times at first. As you improve, you
can do cycles of 5, 10 or more depending on the time you have
and your ability.

Step 5
Return to a neutral hands and knees position and then sit back
into Child's pose to rest.

Side leg lift

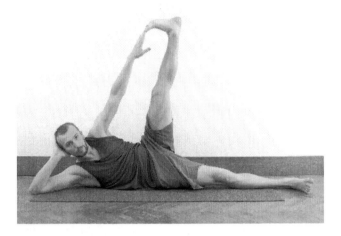

Benefits
- Increases range of motion in the hips
- Firms the buttocks and the backs of the legs
- Increases abdominal and pelvic strength
- Enables sexual positions to be held for longer
- Tones the sides of the torso to reduce "spare tires"

Starting position
Lie on your right side with your right arm under your head. Place your left hand on the floor in front of you. If you feel unsteady you can lie with your back against a wall or some furniture.

Step 1
Lengthen your spine and push out with your heels. Point the fingers of your right hand so that they form a straight line with your neck, spine and legs.

Step 2
Raise your head and bend your right elbow so that you can rest your head in your right palm. Push your elbow along the floor to stretch out your right side and maintain your body's alignment.

Step 3

Point the toes of your left foot towards the ceiling and then draw the left foot towards the pelvis so that it rests about half way along your right leg.

Step 4

Steady yourself then reach your left arm along the inner side of your leg to grab your left big toe as firmly as you can. (If you find this difficult, you can use a belt to loop around your left foot and pull on that instead.)

Step 5

Inhale and pull the left leg straight up towards the ceiling. Avoid rolling your weight backwards or dropping the raised leg forward. Instead try to keep the body aligned as though you were flattened between two panes of glass. Pause and breathe into this position.

Step 6

To release, bring the left foot back to the right knee. Release your grip and stretch the leg out. Use your left arm to push off against the floor and roll onto your back. Bring your right arm alongside the body and rest in Corpse pose.
Repeat on the opposite side.

Camel pose

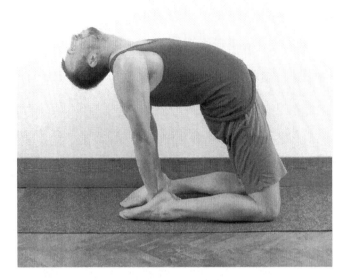

Benefits
- Improves sexual performance through increased stamina and strength
- Improves flexibility right through the body including the pelvis, abdomen and hips
- Stimulates the internal organs and glands and improves their functionality
- Strengthens the back muscles and improves posture
- Opens out the chest and helps to improve respiratory ailments
- Helps to reduce tension and anxiety

Starting position
Kneel on the floor with your knees and ankles hip width apart and the tops of your feet against the floor. Keep your thighs, head and torso in line with each other and at right angles to the floor. It may be useful to visualize an imaginary string just above the crown of your head pulling you in to alignment like a string puppet.

Step 1

Place your hands on your buttocks with the fingers spread and pointing down. Tuck your tailbone in under your pelvis and firm your buttocks to help keep your thighs and spine straight.

Step 2

Raise your right hand and reach to the ceiling with your arm alongside your head then look up at it.

Step 3

With the arm extended, rotate the arm from the shoulder and swing it back and down to grab the right ankle. If you can't reach that far, place the hand on the back of the thigh instead.
While doing this, aim to keep both hips squared to the front and use your left hand and buttocks to push forward and keep the thighs from sagging back.

Step 4

Once you are steady, raise the left arm alongside the head and turn your head to look at the left fingers.

Step 5

Watch your hand as you rotate the left arm back and down. Grab the left ankle and return the head to a neutral position looking up. You can drop the thighs a little to help you reach the left foot or tuck your toes under to raise the heels.

Step 6

Inhale and expand the chest. Aim to bring the thighs and hips forward and straight again. Push into your hands and feet for support. Imagine your puppeteer is now pulling you up from a string attached to your naval so use your abdominal muscles to control the backbend.

Step 7

Allow your head and upper back to drop back loosely and breathe steadily into the lower lungs. Hold this position for a few moments.

Step 8

When you are ready, gently turn your head and look at your left hand. Release the ankle and swing the extended arm up to the ceiling following it with your head.

Step 9
Keeping the left arm up, turn your head and look down at the right hand. Push off from the foot and swing the extended right arm up to the ceiling as you keep looking at the fingers. In the same movement, bring the thighs and hips up and forward to create a straight line between the thighs, torso, head and raised arms.

Step 10
Draw a deep breath and stretch up through the hands and down through the thighs. Then drop both arms to the sides and look to the front. Briefly drop the chin to the chest and extend the back of the neck to release any tension then look forward again.

Step 11
Drop back into Child's pose to reverse the back bend and relax the body. Allow your breathing to return to normal then slowly sit up.

Chapter 9

Fab abs

Poses to strengthen abdominal and lower back muscles

This is possibly one of the reasons you are reading this book right now. Many men want to have a few ripples over a firm abdomen not to mention a firmer backside.

You might also be experiencing back pain or poor posture. The following poses will go a long way to strengthen these areas when performed regularly.

Plank pose
2 variations

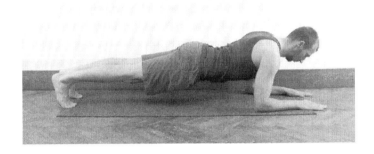

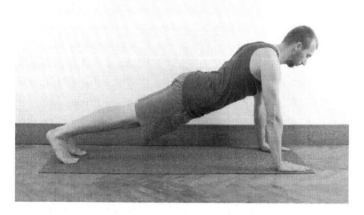

Benefits
- Strengthens the wrists, shoulders, ankles and toes
- Firms the muscles in the arms, abdomen, back and legs
- Improves posture and core strength
- Reduces tension and restores energy

This pose is also sometimes called the "Four-Limbed Staff".

Starting position
Lie on your stomach with your hands by your sides and your head turned to one side

Step 1
Inhale and draw your hands underneath your shoulders and your palms flat on the floor. Spread your fingers wide for greater support. Lift your head up and face the floor.

Step 2
As you exhale, tuck your toes under and tighten your buttocks. Tilt your tailbone towards your heels and draw your abdomen in, pushing any air out of the lower lungs. Lengthen the back of your neck to pull your whole body into a straight line.

Step 3
Inhale and quickly lift your torso off the floor by straightening your arms and pushing with your hands and toes. Keep looking at the floor. Try to keep your spine in line so avoid dropping your hips or raising them too high and lengthen the back of your neck.

As you continue to breathe in deeply try to visualize your ribcage expanding outwards in all directions including sideways.

If you find this position difficult you can rest your elbows and forearms on the floor.

Step 4

To release the position, gently bend your elbows and lower your sternum to the floor. Keep your head and body aligned until the last moment then drop your knees to the floor and untuck your toes.

Give the back of your neck a final stretch by briefly tucking your chin towards your chest, then turn your head to one side and lower it to the floor. Place your arms along your sides with your palms turned up and rest until your breathing returns to normal.

Abdominal lock

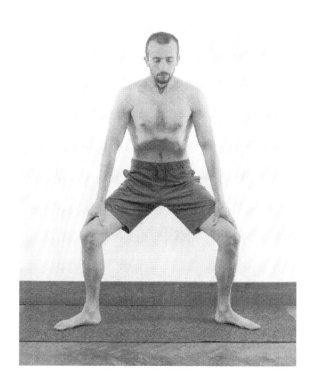

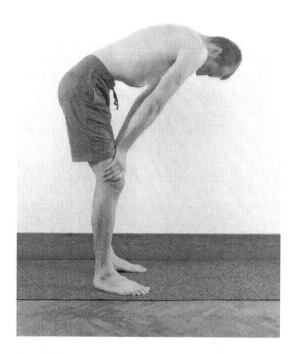

Benefits
- Improves symptoms of indigestion, heartburn and constipation
- Tightens muscles in the abdomen, buttocks and thighs
- Stimulates circulation of blood through the internal organs
- Helps to regulate blood sugar levels
- Strengthens the diaphragm and lower back
- Assists with weight loss
- Helps to balance thyroid fluctuations

Starting position
Begin in Mountain pose

Step 1
Step your legs apart wide and place your hands on the tops of your thighs. Push your tailbone down and pivot your toes outwards but keep your feet flat on the floor.

Step 2
Inhale deeply through your nose into your diaphragm and then quickly exhale through your mouth pushing all your breath out. At the same time, drop into a squat and tuck your chin in to your chest so that you lengthen the back of your neck. Draw your naval in tightly towards your ribs. Aim to keep your thighs parallel to the floor and your spine straight.

   This position will create a lock in both the throat and the groin. Hold without breath for as long as possible (without turning blue).

Step 3
To release, inhale and simply straighten your legs then lift your head and torso upright.
Exhale and drop forward with your fingertips brushing the floor. Look back between your legs and relax your body. Allow your breathing to return to normal.
When you are ready, gradually uncurl your body and step your feet together so you finish in Mountain pose.

Boat pose

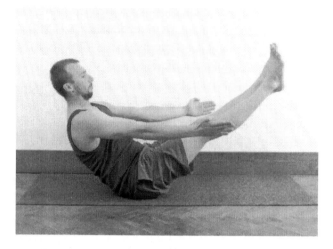

Benefits
- Firms muscles in the back, abdomen, buttocks and legs
- Increases core strength and vitality
- Boosts willpower and determination
- Helps to strengthen lower back and improves hip flexibility
- Improves the function of all internal organs
- Regulates hormonal levels including insulin
- Improves balance and mental focus

Starting position
Sit upright with your legs out in front of you. Bring the knees together and point the toes in the air.

Step 1
Sit with your hands just behind your buttocks and your palms down on the floor. Squeeze your buttocks and shift your weight back so it is distributed evenly between your sitting bones and your tailbone like a tripod.

Step 2
Inhale, then as you exhale draw your knees to the chest and raise your feet off the floor. Keep and your spine straight and avoid hunching your back and neck.

Step 3

Check you are balanced well on your buttocks then raise your arms out in front of you with your elbows straight and your palms facing down. Look straight ahead and pick something stationary to focus on to help you balance. Breathe in this position for a moment.

Step 4

Slowly straighten your legs so they are at around a 45 degree angle to your body. Aim to keep your arms steady and your gaze forward as you do this. Utilize the muscles in your buttocks and abdomen to keep the legs and back straight.

If this pose is too strong for you, you can try keeping your knees bent, holding onto your legs or if needed keep your hands on the floor while you straighten your legs.

Again, pause and hold the position while you breathe into it.

Step 5

Slowly bend your knees and lower your legs into a crossed-legged position. Bring your arms down and stretch them out on the floor in front of you to ease out the spine.

If you lower back is sore, place your feet flat on the floor and hug your knees to your chest, rocking slightly back and forward over your tailbone. You can even hold your knees while you lift your feet off the floor if that feels more comfortable.

Step 6

Undo the position and lie on the floor to rest in Corpse pose.

Chapter 10

Healthy heart heroes

Poses to improve circulation and blood pressure

Our amazing bodies come complete with an internal generator. The humble heart draws oxygen through the lungs and pumps it throughout the body to fuel our billions of cells. It also draws metabolic waste back through the blood to be cleansed and re-oxygenated.

Poor circulation prevents the body from functioning effectively resulting in problems like fatigue, high blood pressure, respiratory issues and varicose veins to name a few.

By actively working to improve circulation we can also take control of our health and reduce the likelihood of future medical issues. Yoga poses such as these have a positive impact on our circulation and heart health. They also help restore general well-being giving us a greater quality of life.

Always remember to come up very slowly after any inverted posture to avoid dizziness or a sudden drop of blood pressure.

Legs up wall

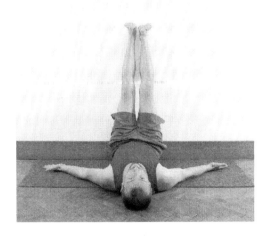

Benefits
- Improves circulation in the legs and feet
- Stabilizes blood pressure
- Helps prevent varicose veins
- Relieves headaches and tension
- Improves digestion and urinary disorders
- Calms the mind and helps with anxiety and mild depression

This pose is an alternative to the Shoulderstand and can be performed any time on its own.

Starting position
Sit with your side close to a free section of wall and your legs straight out in front of you. Place your hands on the floor behind you.

Step 1
Rock back quickly onto your hands and sitting bones, then in one movement, swing both legs up and turn sideways a little so you can place them both against the wall. Your tailbone does not have to be right up against the wall but you should be able to rest both calves against it.

Step 2
Lower your back and head to the floor and spread your arms out to the sides for balance with your palms up. You may like a pillow under your neck or lower back for comfort.

Step 3
Allow your shoulders to roll back and down. Release your thigh and abdominal muscles and close your eyes. As your breathing slows down allow your body to feel heavy as though it is sinking deep into the floor. Stay in this position as long as you like.

Step 4
To come down, draw your knees to your chest, put your right arm up straight beside your ear and use your left hand to help you roll onto your right side.
Stay there for a moment then use your hands to help you roll over onto your hands and knees.

From here you can either sit or stand. Either way, do so slowly and raise your head last of all.

Wedge

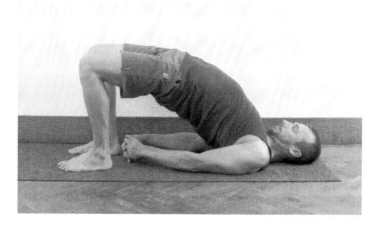

Benefits
- Boosts circulation and regulates blood pressure
- Releases physical and emotional tension
- Stimulates the adrenal and thyroid glands
- Increases lung capacity and improves asthma
- Eases tired legs, back pain and headaches
- Improves flexibility in the spine and strengthens core muscles
- Improves digestion through contraction of the abdominal muscles

Variations include the "Bridge" or "Wheel" poses.

Starting position
Begin in Corpse pose.

Step 1
Inhale then bend your knees and move your feet close to your lower back. If possible, grab hold of your ankles or possibly your trouser legs.

Step 2
Exhale and lift your hips off the floor and clasp your hands

underneath your body. Alternatively, you can bend your elbows and place your hands around your waist to support your torso.

Lift your navel up towards the ceiling and elongate the spine through the backbend. Try to get as high in the pose as you can without straining your neck. It may help to imagine that someone has a string tied to your navel and is pulling it straight up. Feel the body fall naturally back into an arch. Breathe evenly into the lower lungs and hold.

Step 3
Push your belly up slightly then gently lower your back to the floor. To counter the back bend and release any strain, draw your knees to your chest and hug them tight. If you like you can rock your spine slightly against the floor.

Step 4
Straighten your legs and bring your arms back to your sides in Corpse pose.

Downward-facing dog

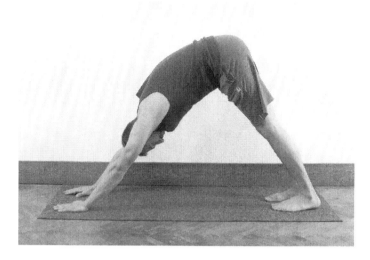

Benefits
- Improves circulation and helps control blood pressure
- Strengthens the joints in the wrists, hands, ankles and feet
- Releases tight muscles in the upper and lower back, hamstrings and calves
- Reduces fatigue and anxiety
- Tones the muscles in the arms and legs

Starting position
Begin on your hands and knees. Keep your wrists below your shoulders and your knees below your hips. Drop your head between your arms and look back to your feet.

Step 1
Spread your palms against the floor, tuck your toes under, then inhale and push your buttocks to the ceiling. Aim to create an upside down "V" shape with your body. Push up with your tailbone and hold the position, breathing steadily into the lower lungs.

Step 2
Come down by dropping your knees to the floor and then swing

your tailbone back and down into Child's pose. Slowly sit up when you are ready.

Chapter 11

Tension busters

Poses to reduce stress and headaches

Sitting or standing for long periods, driving in peak traffic, stressing about finances or dealing with difficult people can all make us extremely tense. Over time this can lead to chronic imbalances in the body causing us pain or sickness.

Simple yoga poses such as these are a drug-free way to restore good health especially when performed regularly.

Cobra pose

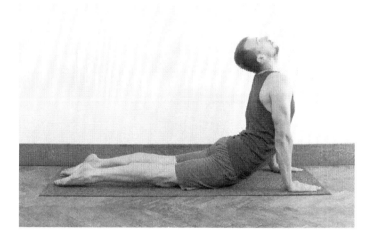

Benefits
- Improves circulation and helps to balance blood pressure
- Releases physical and emotional tension
- Boosts metabolism and energy levels
- Opens out the chest to improve lung function
- Firms muscles in the abdomen, buttocks, thighs and arms
- Helps to relieve back pain and improve suppleness

Starting position
Lie on the floor on your stomach with your head turned to one side and your arms by your sides.

Step 1
Place your hands under each shoulder with the palms down on the floor and your elbows against your sides.

Place your forehead on the floor and point your toes so the tops of the feet touch the floor. Keep your feet close to each other.

Step 2
Inhale then gradually raise your chin and lift your sternum off the floor by pushing with your hands.

Step 3
Continue pushing slowly with your hands as you raise your chest up and arch your back one vertebra at a time. Keep your thighs on the floor and aim to straighten your elbows. Only go as high as you can without forcing it.

For a greater stretch, place your hands alongside your chest before starting to lift.

Imagine that you are a snake slowly waking up and testing the air. You may even gently swing from side to side as though you were responding to a snake charmers music.

Step 4
As you finish your arch, allow your head to rest back between your shoulders and *very* gently squeeze out any tension held there.

Step 5
Hold the position and breathe evenly using your diaphragm to draw air into your lower lungs. Feel your heartbeat become steady.

Step 6
To come out of the position, keep your head dropped back. Instead, draw your abdomen and diaphragm in tight and pull them inwards to uncurl your spine.

At the same time, bend your elbows and very slowly ease your body down until the chest reaches the floor. At the last moment, briefly nod your chin to your chest and then place your head to one side on the floor.

Bring your hands back alongside the body with the palms up

and rest in this position.

Spine twist

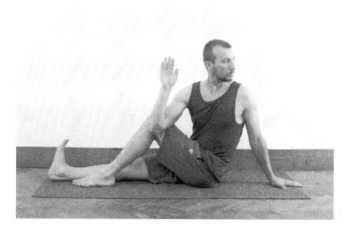

Benefits
- Reduces headaches caused by tight neck muscles
- Eases knots and improves strength in the back muscles
- Generates greater flexibility along the spine
- Improves blood flow to the spinal nerves, veins and tissues
- Reduces physical and emotional tension

Starting position
Sit up with your legs parallel and out in front of you. Point your toes to the ceiling and place your hands on the floor behind your hips.

Step 1
Slide your left foot up until it is flat and alongside the right knee.

Step 2
Breathe in and raise your right arm up straight. Exhale and swing it down and around to grasp the left knee. If you can, try hooking your right elbow around the left knee and placing the right palm along the outside of the left thigh.

Step 3
Inhale and lift your left arm up straight. As you exhale, keep the

elbow straight and swing the arm back and down watching it as it goes. Place the hand flat on the floor just behind the left hip with the fingers pointing away.

Step 4
Twist your chest and shoulders around to the left using your abdominal muscles. Pull upwards through the spine to maintain vertical alignment and avoid sagging into the lower back. Continue to rotate the upper spine while you use your right hand to push against the left leg. Aim to keep your hips and buttocks on the floor and hold the position

Step 5
To come out of the position turn your head to the front then raise your right arm up to the ceiling. Swing it back and down and rest your hand beside the right hip.
Take your left arm and swing it up towards the ceiling, then continue the arc and drop the arm forward and down until your left hand is beside the left hip.
Lower your left knee to the floor and shake your body to release any tension. Repeat the pose on the other side

Wide-angle forward bend

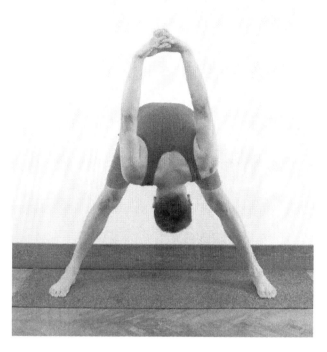

Benefits
- Releases tension held in the back, neck and legs
- Tones the thighs and calves
- Opens out the chest and helps to clear mucus from the lower lungs
- Improves circulation and digestion
- Strengthens the joints and bones
- Reduces fatigue
- Slows the breathing and calms the mind

Starting position
Stand in Mountain pose then step your feet wide apart with your toes pointing inwards.

Step 1
Grasp your hands together behind your back and draw in a deep breath. Use your abdominal and thigh muscles to push the

chest up. Pull up through your crown and tilt your tailbone under the pelvis to extend the spine.

Step 2
Raise your joined hands to the ceiling as you tilt your head and torso forward from the hips. Keep the spine extended and your head between your arms then look back between your legs. Push your hands towards the ceiling to create leverage as you aim to bring your head down further.

Step 3
Hang in this position for as long as you like. When you are ready, push your hands back and down. Keep your head between your arms and your back straight, then pivot from the hips and bring the head and torso upright.
Use your abdominal and thigh muscles and avoid hunching your back as you straighten up.

Step 4
Release your grasp and swing your arms back and up to the ceiling then simply let them drop loosely to your sides.
Step your feet together and rest in Mountain pose.

Chapter 12

Brain training

Poses to improve mental focus and clarity

In our busy lives it's easy to get caught up in so many activities that we feel like we have to juggle them all and not let any slip. While multi-tasking is useful in the short term if we sustain it we often find that nothing ends up getting done properly. Sometimes it is better to sit back and work out what our priorities are. Chose the tasks most important to you and learn to delegate or say "no" to others. These poses will help you focus more deeply on the things that matter and give them 100% of your efforts.
If you have back issues you may find these poses difficult. Try the "Legs up the wall" pose in Chapter 10 instead.

Plow to Shoulder stand

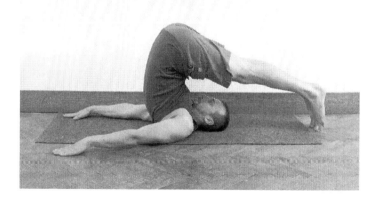

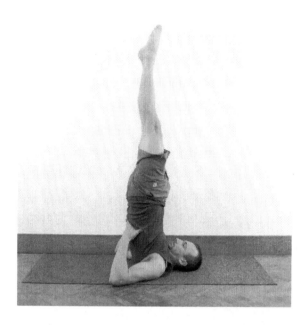

Benefits

- Stimulates cerebral nerves and improves oxygen supply to the brain
- Boosts imagination, intuition and creativity
- "Clears the head" and improves mental clarity and focus
- Balances hormonal activity in the thyroid and prostate glands
- Releases physical and emotional tension and relaxes the body
- Strengthens the neck, shoulders, back, abdomen, buttocks and legs

The Plow pose is a preparation pose for many inversions including the Shoulderstand, Headstand and Handstand. It allows you to get the sensation of standing on your head but with more support. Men are most likely to be able to perform inversions as beginners than women because they naturally have more arm and core strength. Avoid relying on momentum to perform these poses.

Starting position
Begin in Corpse pose and push your knees and ankles together.

Point your toes towards the ceiling.

Step 1
Using your core strength; push your arms against the floor and raise your pelvis and hips up above your chest. Push your tailbone towards the ceiling to extend your spine. Your feet should be touching the floor behind your head or hovering just above it in a reverse forward bend. This is the Plow pose.

Step 2
From Plow pose, you can transition to Shoulderstand by bending your knees and resting them on your forehead

Step 3
Tuck your elbows close to your body and use your hands to support your upper back. Push your feet towards the ceiling and straighten your knees. Try to keep your body in alignment. (This time the puppeteer is pulling you up from your heels.) Hold for as long as you can and breathe steadily.

Step 4
You can release this position by bending your knees to the forehead, laying your arms on the floor for support and gently unrolling the spine until your feet are flat on the floor. Keep your head on the floor as you unwind. Use your buttocks and abdominal muscles to slowly control this movement.

Step 5
Straighten your legs and rest in Corpse pose. Always follow with the Fish pose to counter the back bend. (See Chapter 13.)

Dolphin to headstand

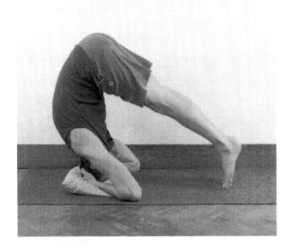

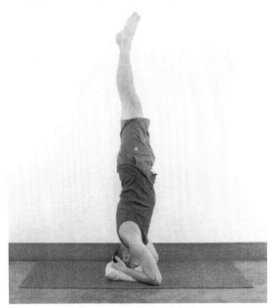

Benefits
- Balances blood pressure and improves oxygen supply to the brain
- Relieves tension and anxiety and may help manage mild depression

- Improves mental focus and clarity
- Strengthens the bones helping to prevent osteoporosis
- Reduces mental and physical sluggishness
- Helps to relieve sciatica, sore feet, insomnia and headaches
- Strengthens and tones muscles throughout the body

Starting position
Begin on your hands and knees with your chin tucked to your chest. If you like you can use a wall for balance so begin with your fingertips touching the wall.

Step 1
Tuck your toes under. Interlace your fingers but leave your elbows on the floor.

Step 2
Raise your buttocks while you lower the crown of your head to the floor between your palms. You may need to adjust your position to find the "flat" spot on the top of your head.

Step 3
Keeping your forearms on the floor push with your toes and straighten your knees so your tailbone is stretched up towards the ceiling and your body forms an upside down "V". This is the Dolphin pose.

Step 4
Keep your weight balanced on the tripod created by your forearms and head. Ensure the back of the neck is not compressed.
Gently walk your feet towards your elbows as far as you can. Continue to push your tailbone up and to hold the pelvis up away from the chest.

Step 5
Once you cannot move your feet closer, pivot from the hips, bend your knees and use your abdominal and back muscles to lift your feet up above your pelvis.
Straighten your knees and push the soles of your feet towards the ceiling to perform a full headstand. Aim to maintain a straight line from your heels down through your knees, hips, shoulders, neck and head. Hold the position.

Step 6

To come down, bend your knees and then place one foot at a time on the floor, returning to Dolphin pose.

Lastly, drop your knees to the floor, release your hands and feet and rest your body in Child's pose. Before standing up, make 2 fists and stack one above the other. Place your forehead on them momentarily to allow your blood pressure to stabilize. Then, keeping your head down, slowly stand up and take a few breaths. Once you are steady, raise your head and finish in Mountain pose.

Teddy bear to Supported headstand

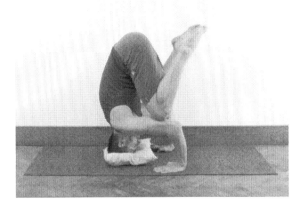

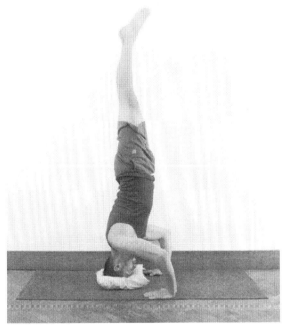

Benefits
- Improves physical and mental balance
- Stimulates cognitive activity and increases creativity
- Improves focus and mental clarity
- Reduces sluggishness throughout the mind and body
- Builds overall strength

- Improves posture
- Strengthens the legs, abdomen, buttocks, arms, shoulders and neck

Starting position
Begin by sitting on your heels with your toes tucked under and your hands on your thighs.

Step 1
Place your hands flat on the floor with your wrists beside your knees and your fingers spread wide. Lift your tailbone away from your heels.

Step 2
Place the crown of your head flat on the floor slightly in front of you so that it forms a triangle with your 2 hands.

Step 3
Lift your buttocks forward and up slightly and check you can balance between your hands and head. Keep your upper arms close to the body and your elbows straight above your wrists.

Step 4
Pushing through your toes, straighten your knees and raise your tailbone to the ceiling so that it is in line above your hips and head.

Step 5
Step your feet forward until your knees rest on the back of your elbows.

Step 6
Carefully bend the right knee and raise the foot until the knee rests on the back of the right elbow.

Step 7
Adjust your balance and then place your left knee onto the back of the left elbow. Push your tailbone and heels towards the ceiling and keep your feet together.
This is the Teddy Bear pose or Half Headstand. Once you are balanced you can hold this position as it is usually quite comfortable.

Step 8
Move to a full headstand by engaging the core muscles and pushing the heels up to the ceiling as you straighten your legs. Keep your weight balanced between your head and hands and work to keep your pelvis from sinking onto your chest.

Step 9
Release the pose by extending first one leg and then the other to the floor. Return to your hands and knees then sit back in Child's pose briefly.

Step 10
Form 2 fists and place one on top of the other. Raise your buttocks, swing your torso forward and place your forehead down on the fist stack. Rest like this while your heart rate and breathing return to normal.

Step 11
When you are ready, slowly stand but leave your head dropped down until your body is upright. Finally lift your chin and stand in Mountain pose.

Chapter 13

Chill out man

Poses for relaxation

To wind down after a busy day or to relieve pain and tension nothing beats these soothing poses. Create a few minutes of uninterrupted time in a quiet space and allow your body the opportunity to recharge.

Tension builds up over time so we often don't notice it. However by practicing regular relaxation you will soon notice a huge difference in your energy and physical comfort.

The ultimate relaxation position is the Corpse pose. Here are some others you may also enjoy.

Fish pose

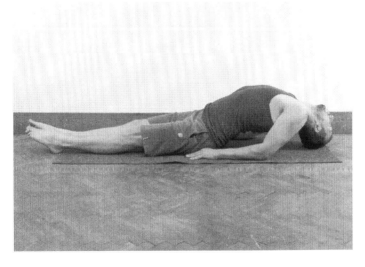

Benefits
- Calms the breath and reduces anxiety

- Helps to relieve neck pain and headaches
- Stretches and tones the muscles of the neck and face
- Expands the bronchial tubes and improves respiratory issues
- Balances the function of the thyroid, pineal, pituitary and adrenal glands

The Fish and the Shoulderstand normally form a mini-sequence; however the Fish can also be done on its own.

Starting position
Lie in Corpse pose and place your palms on the floor.

Step 1
Tuck your hands under your buttocks and place your thumbs and index fingers on either side of your sitting bones in a "V" shape.

Step 2
Push your elbows under your chest and pull your upper torso to the ceiling leading with your solar plexus. (The puppeteer has you again.)

As your chest lifts, bring your shoulder blades together and allow your head to follow until your crown rests lightly on the floor.

Take your weight on your forearms and extend your lower body, pointing the toes away. Breathe deeply into your lower lungs and hold the position.

Step 3
To come down, inhale and gently lift your head a fraction then as you exhale pull your diaphragm down and gently uncurl your spine. At the last moment stretch the back of your neck out and rest your head on the floor.

Step 4
Straighten your legs and return to Corpse pose. If you are not doing a shoulder stand counter this pose by hugging your knees and curling your head to your chest in a fetal position momentarily.

Forward bend with folded arms

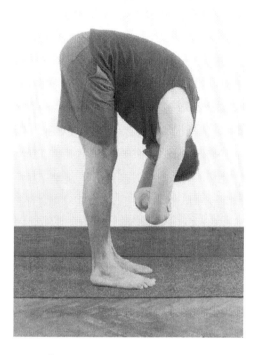

Benefits
- Soothes the nervous system
- Reduces physical and emotional tension
- Slows the breathing and a racing mind
- Eases back pain
- Improves posture
- Stretches and tones the calves and hamstrings

Starting position
Begin in Mountain pose.

Step 1
Inhale and reach your hands up towards the ceiling.

Step 2
Exhale and lean forward and down keeping your arms, head and back in alignment and pivoting from the hips. Push your tailbone

back as a counter-balance.

Step 3
Continue to lower yourself until your arms dangle towards your feet and push your tailbone up towards the ceiling.

Step 4
Grasp each elbow with the opposite hand and let your head hang loose so you can look back between your knees. Keep your heels on the floor and feel the stretch down the back of your legs.

Feel the weight of your arms stretch out your back and neck muscles. Let your breathing slow down and allow your thoughts to lose focus. Close your eyes and visualize any tension dripping down from your body.

Step 5
Unfold your arms and place your hands on your shins. Come up very gradually by uncurling the spine, keeping your head down and sliding your hands up to your knees. Pause in a gentle squat before standing straight up. Finally lift your head and stand in Mountain pose.

Child's pose

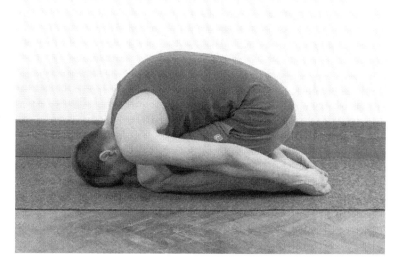

Benefits
- Greatly reduces tension and muscular pain
- Calms the mind and helps relieve stress and anxiety
- Reduces fatigue
- Improves mental focus
- Strengthens the spine, hips, thighs and ankles
- Improves circulation and regulates blood pressure
- Increases flexibility throughout the body

Starting position
Begin on your hands and knees with the tops of the feet against the floor and your heels out to the sides. Touch your big toes together. You may need to place a rolled towel or blanket on top of your feet as a support for your tailbone.

Step 1
Push your hands forward on the floor palms down. Lower your chest and keep your head between your elbows. As you do this, push your tailbone back and down between your heels, sitting on the rolled towel if needed.

Step 2
Let the chest rest on the thighs and if possible, drop your forehead to the floor.

If you find this difficult, create 2 fists and stack one above the other. Allow your forehead to rest on them instead.

Step 3
Close your eyes then either keep your arms stretched forward with your palms on the floor or bring them to your sides with palms up and your fingers pointing towards your feet.

Step 4
Allow your body to rest deeply in this position. With each exhalation let any tension melt away. Stay in this pose for as long as you want to.

Step 5
When you are ready, very slowly uncurl your spine and sit up on your heels with your hands on your thighs and your chin on your chest.

From here you can either stand up or swing your legs to the front and sit in a comfortable position.

Give the back of your neck a final stretch then use your abdominal muscles to help lift the head back to a neutral position. Open your eyes and give your body a little shake to wake yourself up.

Conclusion

I hope this book was able to help you understand the benefits of yoga and learn the basic postures quickly and easily.

Adding yoga into your daily life can be very simple as you can see it can only take minutes a day, you can start straight away and begin enjoying the many benefits.

The next step is to get your mat out and get your OM on. Follow the easy steps outlined in this book and be on your way to becoming a full-fledged yogi.

Finally, if you enjoyed this book, then I'd like to ask you for a favor, would you be kind enough to leave a review for this book on Amazon? It'd be greatly appreciated! Thank you and good luck!

Further Reading

Yoga For Beginners - A Simple Guide To A Slim Body, Stress Relief And Inner Peace by Nicole Talbot

- An excellent introduction to Yoga for Beginners
Corewalking.com
- An excellent website with multiple articles explaining how the human body moves.

Yoga for Fibromyalgia

- This video provides yoga tips for anyone with chronic pain or stiffness

Meditation for beginners

- A great site for those who want to explore relaxation and meditation further

Made in the USA
San Bernardino, CA
08 February 2016